Successful Battle in Treating Low Back Pain with Herbal Remedies

Natural Pain Management

I0447253

Guy Chamberland, M.Sc., Ph.D., Master Herbalist

Disclaimer

Prior to taking any new herbal products/supplements, always check with your health-care practitioner.

ISBN 978-1477539750

DEDICATION

To my wife, Céline, who gave me the opportunity to learn and practice herbology, and to my four daughters Elodie, Min Jee, Clara and Laura-Marie.

TABLE OF CONTENTS

INTRODUCTION

Guy Chamberland was first introduced to Chinese herbal medicine in 1990. This launched his interest in herbal medicine, and over the years he studied the pharmacology of many herbs.

Based on his experience working on complex pharmaceutical products, he was invited to present at the FDA Public Hearing on Regulation of Combination Products (http://www.fda.gov/CombinationProducts/Meet-ingsConferencesWorkshops/ucm133825.htm).

Subsequently he wrote a chapter entitled "*Developing Drug-Device Combination Products with Unapproved Components*" for the textbook **Clinical Evaluation of Medical Devices**, edited by Becker, Karen M. and Whyte, John J., Humana Press, 2006.

In 2007 Guy Chamberland began studying the additive and synergistic effects obtained when combining plant extracts. His interest in herbal pain management began early in 2007 after suffering from a L4-L5 disc hernia. This book is about how he successfully treated this condition using herbal remedies.

In 2009 Guy Chamberland founded a company called CuraPhyte Technologies Inc. (www.curaphyte.com; www.enteriphyte.com) that specializes in the development and commercialization of evidence-based herbal remedies. The company has two major axes of activities: one devoted to commercializing quality products for patient self-care lines, and the other devoted to commercializing professional product lines and working closely with health practitioners to further understand the treatment of pain with herbal remedies.

Guy Chamberland has completed training as a natural health practitioner, bioenergetics practitioner, chartered herbalist, in herbal prescriptions, and performed clinical research to obtain the degree of Master Herbalist. Through his continued research in herbal science, he has become an expert in herbal pain management.

Chapter 1
MEDICAL CONDITION: DISC HERNIA

One morning in May 2007, he was seated writing away on a computer and everything changed when he stood up to go get a cup of coffee. He went from a healthy condition to being a patient with a disc hernia at L4-L5. He rapidly discovered the world of pain and had never imagined that in 2012 he would still face challenges of chronic pain from the disc hernia.

The symptoms consisted of pain radiating from the lower back all the way to the tip of the toes. On a scale of 0 to 10 the intensity of the pain ranged from 8 to 10 depending on the daily activities. Simple tasks, such as putting socks on or tying a shoe lace, became a daily challenge. He could not bend over to put on socks or tie shoe laces. Lying on his side or sitting on the floor was the only way he could put his socks on or tie a shoe lace.

A 10 kilogram object was too heavy to lift without worsening the level of pain. No jumping or running was possible. On a daily basis, the lower leg muscle cramps, which were like a tight knot in the leg, stopped him from walking and forced him to sit or lay down. There was numbness on the surface of the skin of the right thigh.

The pain prevented him from falling asleep. Any body movement resulted in pain and kept him awake at night. Sexual activity always resulted in severe pain.

Getting out of bed had its unique sensations. Some mornings, after waking up, a significant part of the pain was gone. However, getting out of bed and walking would launch another day where the pain would gradually grow in intensity and reach its maximum at night.

Tylenol® and/or Motrin® did not provide any degree of pain relief. Four milligrams of hydromorphone was not sufficient to remove the pain. Nothing helped reduce the severe muscle cramping.

After several days of enduring the severe pain and sleepless nights, it was time to discover the cause and seek professional medical help.

A Magnetic Resonance scan and CAT scan were performed and revealed the following diagnosis. The spinal column canal was found to be small based on short pedicles. This was of congenital origin. At L3-L4 there was a slight diffuse spreading disc with anterior spondylosis and loss of posterior concavity. At L4-L5 there was central disc herniation causing a mild to moderate reduction of the caliber of the spinal canal.

The 4 mg of hydromorphone were complemented with 500 mg Naprosyn® and 10 mg Flexeril®. This cocktail provided good relief but made him completely non-functional. The undesirable side effects, including drowsiness, loss of concentration, uncoordinated motor skills, etc., prevented him from continuing his scientific research. The use of these medications was definitely not something he wanted. The desire to return to a functional mental and physical life meant getting off these medications. Addiction to a narcotic was not an issue. This cocktail made him feel like a vegetable and this was not an acceptable alternative; especially as a father with small children. The treating physician had little interest in the impact of the medications on the quality of life. His only comment was that with time his body would get used to these adverse effects. It was this comment that triggered the quest for a non-addictive and non-vegetable-inducing remedy. These drugs were not the path he wanted.

The medical specialist recommended surgery. Guy Chamberland was against this approach but took time to consider the options. Pending surgery, the physician prescribed 3 treatments, one month apart, with epidural injections of a local anesthetic plus corticosteroids. This treatment only caused partial pain relief that lasted not more than a week. The injections resulted in facial flushing, severe hypertension and aggressiveness. He informed the physician that he would not go for the third injection as this therapy did not provide sufficient pain relief to justify the adverse effects.

The next visit with the medical specialist was the last. His decision was made. The lack of pharmaceutical drugs that could relieve the pain, and allow him to actively work as a scientist, led to the decision to turn to alternative medicine. Surgery was not an acceptable alternative for him; especially without having tried herbal remedies.

This motivated Dr. Chamberland's research into the development of herbal based remedies for pain. Why was he so confident that he could find herbs to treat this condition?

In 1990, he was introduced to Traditional Chinese medicine. After several years of antimicrobial drug therapies, his physicians concluded that conventional medicine had no cure for a persistent pulmonary infection. His next book is entitled *Scientific Look at Herbal Remedies: Is there more than Traditional Evidence*? It will discuss this pulmonary condition in more detail as well as provide an objective look at the evidence backing the traditional use of herbs in the treatment of many health conditions.

After several weeks of taking infusions of a Chinese herb, the pulmonary infection was gone and Guy Chamberland's pulmonary medical specialist stated: it shows that they have been practicing medicine for over 5000 years.

After being cured by an herbal remedy in 1990 and with many years of experience developing new drugs for the pharmaceutical industry, it was clear to him that herbs could be used to create remedies that were as strong as pain relief drugs (e.g. anti-inflammatory, analgesic).

In 2007, several months after making the decision not to undergo surgery, he began taking a blend of anti-inflammatory herbs. The switch was done from conventional pharmaceutical drugs to herbal remedies. These herbs had both anti-inflammatory and analgesic properties. Five years later in 2012, he still has on a daily basis a sensation of pain in his big toe. Moderate-to-severe pain results after any false movement, lifting a heavy object, or physical exertion involving the lower back. Anti-inflammatory and antispasmodic herbs are immediately used and at night an analgesic and sedative herb is taken for night pain and pain-related insomnia.

Herbal remedies have allowed Guy Chamberland to avoid surgery and have an excellent quality of life despite the chronic pain and challenges of a persistent disc hernia. These herbs are at least as strong as the prescription drugs used but without the negative side effects or risk of physical dependence.

The next chapters will describe the use of these herbs to treat severe pain and manage pain-induced conditions like insomnia. This book is not a textbook on herbal pain management. It is about how he used these remedies to successfully battle chronic low back pain and its pain-related conditions. For a complete book on herbal pain management, read Guy Chamberland's textbook entitled: *The Use of Herbal Remedies in the Treatment of Pain*.

Chapter 2
HERBAL PAIN MANAGEMENT

There are four key treatment aspects to the management of pain from disc hernias and the consequences caused by the pain, such as insomnia. These are anti-inflammatory, analgesic, antispasmodic and sedative (hypnotic) herbs.

The anti-inflammatory herbs are the main treatment to reduce the inflammation and pain and maintain the pain reduction. These should be the base therapy and need to be taken daily to ensure adequate reduction of the inflammation and pain. The usage should be decreased as the pain evolves and the pain is reduced.

The analgesic herbs are also critical to reduce the pain when it is unbearable, especially at night. It is important to also view analgesics as rescue therapy for when the pain becomes intolerable.

Antispasmodic herbs should only be used in conditions when there are muscle cramps or spasms. Therefore, these are remedies to use as needed. However, do not use more per day than recommended by the manufacturer unless directed by a healthcare practitioner.

Pain-related insomnia is a major issue for patients with disc hernias. There are some herbs that are both analgesic and sedative and these can be used successfully to reduce pain and allow the patient to sleep. There are other herbs that are sedative and can be used in combination with the analgesic herbs to obtain a stronger sedative action.

In 2007, Guy Chamberland switched from prescription drugs to herbal remedies. The pharmaceutical drugs taken were Naprosyn™ (anti-inflammatory), Dilaudid™ (analgesic), and Flexiril™ (muscle relaxant). These were replaced with a blend of anti-inflammatory and analgesic herbs. As recommended by an herbalist (a colleague of Guy Chamberland's with over 20 years of clinical practice), the first two days he took twice the recommended dosage. Subsequently, he used the recommended daily dosage.

The herbs worked very well in reducing the pain and on most days there was no need to use a rescue analgesic to relieve excessive pain. On occasion, after a false movement or exertion the pain was unbearable and rescue analgesia was needed. In 2007, he had not yet developed adequate herbal analgesics and used Dilauid™ as rescue therapy. In 2009, he developed an expertise in analgesic herbs and from that point there was no need for any non-herbal rescue therapies, such as Dilauid™.

He faced the same issue with muscle spasms and cramps. Prior to 2009, Guy Chamberland used Flexeril™ to reduce the lower leg cramping and muscle spasms. As of 2009 this pharmaceutical drug was successfully replaced with antispasmodic herbs.

Over the years he developed the habit of viewing herbs as being equivalent to the pharmaceutical drugs. Some people have a bottle of acetaminophen and/or ibuprofen on the pharmacy shelf for emergency pain relief. He has herbs and turns to herbs for severe pain and muscle cramps and spasms. You also find sedative herbs on his shelf for insomnia.

The anti-inflammatory herbs were taken twice daily over more than 1 year. It basically took this time for the body to 'repair' the herniated disc. On occasion there were severe flare ups and the dosage of the herbs was doubled until the pain intensity returned to the pre-flare up level.

Part of the recovery involves learning how to live with the disc hernia. Certain activities (e.g. lifting heavy objects, running) or a false movement can result in mild-to-severe pain flare ups. The level of pain intensity is what lets you know when to increase the daily dosage. This 'doubling' of the daily dosage was explained by the herbalist and it became a habit of living with the pain.

After approximately 1.5 years of taking anti-inflammatory herbs daily, he was able to stop daily use. He initially had to be careful with what to lift or what activities to perform. However, the body quickly learns what it can do not to induce moderate-to-severe pain. During this time, he often turned to the herbs as rescue therapies.

The muscle relaxant drug was replaced with an antispasmodic herb. This herb was used when the lower leg cramping or spasms would begin. It was also used in combination with the anti-inflammatory herbs after exertion to rapidly reduce the lower back pain and muscular spasms.

Pain tends to increase during the day and by night it is at its maximal level. To obtain quality and restorative sleep, Guy Chamberland took an analgesic herb that was both a sedative and analgesic. This combination allowed the use of one product only and it worked very well.

Other than the high level of efficacy obtained from the herbs, the major difference versus the prescription drugs was the quality of life. He did not have any side effects from the herbs. There was no risk of drug addiction or physical dependence and there was no next morning residual sedative effect, no constipation, no motor incoordination and none of the side effects common with narcotics, such as lack of concentration, decreased memory, aggressiveness, etc. He felt like a 'vegetable' taking the pharmaceutical cocktail and could not work. With the herbs, he felt like a fully functional person and could both work and enjoy life.

Living with pain does not mean that there is no pain or that pain flare ups do not occur. It means that you learn how to self-treat certain aspects of the pain on a daily basis allowing you to have a high quality of life. He learned what to take rapidly after the first signs of increasing pain begin or when muscle spasms or cramping begin.

Over the years Guy Chamberland developed a tolerance to the daily sensation of pain in the toes. Some days he prefers not feeling the pain so he takes anti-inflammatory herbs in the morning. Most of the time he tolerates the pain and only turns to herbal remedies when the lower back pain or when muscle spasms begin.

He does not let the insomnia impact his quality of life. He commonly turns to herbs to fall and stay asleep. These remedies are taken at the first sign that he cannot fall asleep. This is an acceptable approach since the herbs have no side effects commonly associated with a sleep aid drug. There is no point in thinking about falling asleep for hours. The chapter on insomnia will explain the use of herbs for obtaining a restful sleep and staying asleep.

Chapter 3
MANAGEMENT OF INFLAMMATION

This chapter introduces the reader to some strong anti-inflammatory herbs and to those Guy Chamberland used and still uses to reduce the pain from a chronic disc hernia. It then discusses the use of these herbs for the treatment of low back pain from disc hernias.

Black currant (*Ribes nigrum*) is commonly used in Europe as an anti-inflammatory remedy. The active anti-inflammatory part of the plant *Ribes nigrum* is the leaves. Doses range from 2 to 4 grams of dried leaves taken orally several times a day. According to van Wyk & Wink (2010), remedies made from the leaves were used to treat arthritis, rheumatism, spasmodic cough and diarrhea. Guy Chamberland has used this herb as an anti-inflammatory ingredient since 2007. Combined with some of the other herbs it was effective in relieving pain.

Boswellia (*Boswellia sacra or serrata*), also known as Frankincense tree, is well known for its anti-inflammatory and analgesic properties. The active part of the plant is the resin. The inhibition of 5-lipoxygenase has been proposed as a path for its beneficial effects in arthritis. Some products use this herbal agent as an anti-inflammatory and analgesic remedy. He has used this herb for the management of other pain conditions and in topical products for both its anti-inflammatory and analgesic properties.

Devil's claw (*Harpagophytum procumbens*) is a South African plant that is recognized for its anti-inflammatory properties. The active part of the plant is the dried secondary roots. It is considered a bitter tonic and an anti-inflammatory, antirheumatic and analgesic remedy. Doses range from 0.6 to 9 grams of the dried root daily and can be taken as infusions (or the equivalent in the form of a dried extract) of 1 to 3 grams per dose. Today it is very popular for its use in the treatment of rheumatism and arthritis. Guy Chamberland uses this herb in many products for the treatment of pain and inflammation and especially in the treatment of pain due to disc hernias. His clinical studies demonstrated that both alone, and in combination with other herbs, Devil's claw is a very effective anti-inflammatory remedy. He has had great results using this herb in combination with the analgesic herb California poppy (*Eschscholzia californica*) and antispasmodic herb Scullcap (*Scutellaria lateriflora*).

There have been over 20 clinical trials with Devil's claw showing benefits to low back pain, osteoarthritis and rheumatoid arthritis. The iridoid glycosides (e.g. harpagoside) have been linked to its anti-inflammatory and analgesic benefits.

Feverfew (*Chrysanthemum parthenium*) is a well-known herb for its benefits in the prevention of migraine headaches. The active parts of the plant are the aerial parts. It has been traditionally used to treat migraine, fever, rheumatic and skin conditions as well as gynaecological disorders (van Wyk & Wink 2010). Doses range from 50 to 200 mg of dried leaves per day. Some research studies have demonstrated its anti-inflammatory properties. Some herbalists add it to products to obtain this benefit.

Figwort (*Scrophularia nodosa*), also known as **Common Figwort**, has been overlooked as a remedy for the treatment of pain and other conditions. The active plant parts are the dried aerial parts. It used to be well known for its anti-inflammatory and analgesic properties. Doses range from 2 to 8 grams of the dried herb taken as an infusion or equivalent quantities in forms of extracts or tinctures taken daily. Guy Chamberland uses this herb for mild-to-moderate knee pain. It is a very good herb for reducing swelling and inflammation of the joints, such as the knee.

This herb contains several iridoid glycosides including harpagoside, harpagide, aucubin, catapol and procumbide giving it a composition similar to that of Devil's claw. Some of these ingredients have well established anti-inflammatory properties.

Horsetail (*Equisetum arvense*), also known as **Field Horsetail**, is an herb commonly used in North America, Europe and Asia for its diuretic effects (van Wyk & Wink 2010). The active part of the plant is the dried stems and according to van Wyk & Wink (2010), it is used "as a diuretic to treat inflammation of the lower urinary tract, kidney gravel and post-traumatic and static oedema". Doses range from 2 to 6 grams of the dried herb per day. This plant is well known as a source of silicon since it contains 5-8% silicic acid (van Wyk & Wink 2010). Guy Chamberland uses this herb, in combination with other herbs, to effectively treat arthritic pain and low back pain.

Turmeric (*Curcuma longa*) is a well-known herb in India where it is believed to have originated. The active part of the plant is the rhizomes and it is used for its anti-inflammatory properties. Doses range from 2 to 9 grams of the dried rhizome daily. Curcuminoids are recognized for their anti-inflammatory properties. Although Turmeric appears in earlier material medica textbooks (Culbreth 1927), the pain management benefits of this herb were not recognized during this period. Guy Chamberland uses this herbal agent in combination with others to make effective anti-inflammatory remedies. It is also used by herbalists for its protective effects to the gastrointestinal tract and liver.

The anti-inflammatory activity is dependent on the dose of the herbal ingredient. When used at the adequate dosage, some herbal ingredients are sufficiently strong anti-inflammatory agents to be used alone. In these cases, the product will provide pain relief just like a prescription Non-Steroidal Anti-Inflammatory Drug (NSAID) does. Guy Chamberland uses an enteric coated tablet containing a standardized extract of the secondary root of Devil's claw. The enteric coating is essential because it has been scientifically demonstrated that the active ingredients of Devil's claw are degraded in the stomach by acid hydrolysis. The enteric coated formulation of Devil's claw contains an adequate amount of the extract to provide pain relief in conditions like arthritis and low back pain due to disc hernias. This product was tested in a clinical trial in patients with moderate-to-severe acute pain as assessed on a Visual Analog Scale (VAS). This study demonstrated significant pain relief in patients that took two enteric coated tablets of Devil's claw, twice a day, along with California poppy (once at night) and Scullcap (2 tablets three times a day).

Guy Chamberland commonly uses standardized extracts to ensure that each batch/lot of remedy is of comparable strength. This is important for making a quality product but also for patients wanting the same benefit day-to-day.

Beginning in 2007, he performed research using experimental models of acute and chronic pain and inflammation. This research led to the understanding of which herbs worked in combination, in an additive or synergistic relationship. He used this knowledge to create strong anti-inflammatory blends of herbal agents. There are several products on the market that are well designed in terms of herbal ingredients and amount of the ingredients. One product consists of a combination of Devil's claw, Black currant, Turmeric, Horsetail and omega-3 fatty acids. The latter ingredient is from fish oil. His research demonstrated that omega-3 fatty acids worked very well in combination with these ingredients. A clinical trial in patients demonstrated that this herbal product was effective in reducing pain and inflammation in patients. In this trial, patients with chronic moderate-to-severe pain (assessed using a VAS) took this blend of anti-inflammatory herbs, two capsules three times a day, along with a blend of Devil's claw and California poppy at night. The study demonstrated significant pain relief and improvements in mobility. Guy Chamberland also uses this product as an alternative to pharmaceutical NSAIDs when strong anti-inflammatory activity is required.

The significant advantage of the enteric coated Devil's claw product is that the harpagoside active ingredients are protected from degradation in the stomach and therefore patients will obtain adequate pain relief. In the case of the multi-herbal anti-inflammatory ingredient product, it is not enteric coated so degradation of active ingredients like harpagoside is possible if you eat just before or while taking the product. However, the product contains a sufficient quantity of other anti-inflammatory ingredients to provide adequate pain relief and inhibition of the inflammation pathways.

He uses either of the above anti-inflammatory products to relieve the pain caused by the disc hernia. When the pain is severe he may have to take the products for several days along with the antispasmodic and analgesic herbs.

You can learn more about the products Guy Chamberland develops for pain relief, and pain-associated insomnia, by visiting his website at www.guy-chamberland-herbalist.com. From this website you will find links to the different product brands that are based on his research.

Chapter 4

ANALGESIC HERBS FOR PAIN

This chapter introduces the reader to analgesic herbs and to those Guy Chamberland used and still uses to reduce the pain from a chronic disc hernia. It then discusses the use of these herbs for the treatment of low back pain from disc hernias.

Black cohosh (*Cimicifuga racemosa*), also known as **Black snakeroot**, has a long history of use with Native Indians in the treatment of pain and menstrual disorders. The active parts of the plant are the dried rhizome and roots. Doses range from 0.4 to 2.4 grams of the dried rhizome and/or root per day.

It was first used as a medicine in 1831 for the treatment of rheumatism, neuralgia, dysmenorrhea, as well as other non-pain conditions (Culbreth 1927). The medicinal drug Macrotys was prepared from the plant Black cohosh and was launched in Eclectic medicine in 1844 as a remedy for acute rheumatism and neuralgia (Felter 1922). It had many clinical indications for use including the treatment of rheumatoid and myalgic pain (Felter 1922). Over time, it developed a reputation as an excellent remedy/anodyne (relieves pain) for rheumatoid pain (Felter 1922; Ellingwood & Lloyd 1919). This medicine was thought to possess sedative, cardiac, anodyne and antispasmodic properties. Guy Chamberland uses this herb for the treatment of arthritic pain, menstrual disorders and several none pain conditions. He has developed products using this herb with Common Figwort. His research has demonstrated that this blend is ideal for arthritic conditions with swollen joints and for fibrositis and pain associated with neuralgia (such as sciatica).

Boswellia (*Boswellia sacra or serrata*), also known as Frankincense tree, is well known for its anti-inflammatory and analgesic properties. The active part of the plant is the resin. The inhibition of 5-lipoxygenase has been proposed as a path for its beneficial effects in arthritis. Although this is a very good herb, Guy Chamberland has only used it for pain relief in topical products. It is found in some of his ointments and creams for pain relief due to burns or post-surgical wound healing, for cracked skin, and other skin conditions.

California poppy (*Eschscholzia californica*) is an herb traditionally used in North America for its analgesic, hypnotic and sedative properties. The active part of the plant is the dried aerial parts. Doses range from 0.5 to 3 grams per day of the dried herb. Guy Chamberland observed a dose-response relationship for its pharmacological effects (e.g. analgesia, sedation).

It has been traditionally used to treat sleeplessness (e.g. insomnia) in adults and children, anxiety, minor nervous disturbances, neuralgic pains, toothaches, and liver and gallbladder complaints (van Wyk & Wink 2010). Guy Chamberland uses this herb extensively as an analgesic and sedative. He has developed multiple products with this herb.

You must use this herb wisely as it is powerful when used at an adequate dosage. You may experience drowsiness when taking this herb. In the morning, or during the day, if taking this herb, be very careful if you are using heavy machinery, driving a motor vehicle or involved in activities requiring mental alertness.

It is also a safe herb in that there are no reports of

addiction, physical dependence, constipation, reduced concentration or reduced motor coordination. Basically, none of the side effects typical of a narcotic have been observed, or associated, with this herb. The only reported side effects are drowsiness, altered dreams and insomnia. The insomnia occurs in a very small number of people and this side effect is well-known for the type of activity associated with this herb. The altered dreams are usually pleasant or strange dreams and not nightmares. It is used as a remedy for treating nightmares.

Other experimental studies have confirmed the following pharmacological properties of California poppy (Gafner et al 2006; Rolland et al 2001): sedative, spasmolytic, anxiolytic and analgesic activities. There are no studies or reports suggesting that a person can develop physical dependence or addiction to California poppy. This is why it is not classified as a narcotic or controlled drug.

Meadowsweet (*Filipendula ulmaria*), also known as **queen-of-the-meadow**, is an herb commonly used in Europe and Asia for treating pain. The pharmaceutical drug Aspirin™ was named after *Spiraea ulmaria* which is the old name for Meadowsweet (van Wyk & Wink 2010). The active part of the plant that is traditionally used is the dried flower or dried aerial part of the plant. Remedies made from this plant are considered both anti-inflammatory and analgesic.

Meadowsweet remedies are used in the treatment of arthritis and rheumatism as well as colds for its antipyretic (e.g. reduce fever) properties (van Wyk & Wink 2010). Doses range from 2.5 to 3.5 grams of the dried flower or 4 to 5 grams of the dried herb per day. During the first two years, Guy Chamberland used this herb as an analgesic agent to reduce the pain.

White Willow (*Salix alba*) is a species of willow native to Europe and Asia and is well known for its content of the active ingredient salicin. The active plant part is the dried willow bark from 2 to 3 year old branches (van Wyk & Wink 2010). Doses range from 2 to 3 grams of powdered bark in one cup of cold water and then heating to boiling. A cupful is taken 3 to 4 times per day.

This plant is well known for its anti-inflammatory, analgesic and antipyretic effects. Remedies have traditionally been used for the treatment of fever/flu, rheumatism, headaches and other minor pain. In the early 1900's, its use in treating acute rheumatism, fever, relieving pain, and neuralgia was recognized in the *Manual of Materia Medica* (Culbreth 1927). Guy Chamberland used this herb during the first two years to relieve pain.

The analgesic activity of these herbal agents is dependent on the dosage taken. When used at an adequate dosage, these herbal ingredients are sufficiently strong analgesic agents to be used alone. In these cases, the product will provide pain relief just like acetaminophen or a weak narcotic. Some of these herbs also have anti-inflammatory activity. Aspirin is a Non-Steroidal Anti-Inflammatory Drug (NSAID) so it is normal that Meadow-sweet has anti-inflammatory activity.

Meadowsweet and White Willow are both associated with side effects (Natural Standard database). Meadowsweet contains salicylate ingredients, so adverse effects associated with salicylates can occur (e.g. gastric and renal irritation, hypersensitivity, nausea and vomiting, and tinnitus). Willow bark extract is associated various gastrointestinal side effects, headaches, and allergic reactions. A relatively safer approach is using these two herbs in combination with other herbs. This approach is based on the use of lower levels of each ingredient and that each ingredient will act additively to provide the same relief that a therapeutic dose of the single herb would provide. During the first two years of treatment, Guy Chamberland used an herbal blend containing anti-inflammatory and analgesic herbs. His research had demonstrated that the analgesic herbs would work additively with the anti-inflammatory herbs to reduce the pain.

In 2009, he stopped using these analgesic ingredients and began using California poppy as an analgesic for low back pain. This herb had a much safer profile and was a powerful analgesic. The switch to California poppy brought an additional clinical benefit: sedation. Insomnia is commonly associated with low back pain from disc hernias. California poppy was taken for both its analgesic and sedation benefits. He uses it mainly at night to avoid drowsiness when driving or while at work. Obtaining restful sleep at night was a welcomed benefit especially without fear of developing physical dependence or becoming addicted to the herb.

Guy Chamberland uses both enteric coated tablets and capsules containing extracts of the dried herb top of California poppy. He uses either non-standardized and standardized extracts in the products he develops. The standardized extract of California poppy is used in products developed as strong analgesics and sedatives. The extract used is standardized to three benzylisoquinoline alkaloids. These alkaloids possess the analgesic, sedative and anxiolytic activity of the herb.

Guy Chamberland has performed controlled and uncontrolled clinical studies in patients with pain and/or insomnia. These studies demonstrated the clinical benefit of the herb in the treatment of pain and management of insomnia. A single capsule or tablet of California poppy was taken at night along with anti-inflammatory and antispasmodic herbs as described in other chapters of this book.

Anti-inflammatory agents are sometimes called analgesics because these ingredients relieve pain. The base treatment for the pain caused by the disc hernia is the anti-inflammatory herbs. You could state that the California poppy is providing co-analgesia when both types of herbal products are used in combination. The sedation obtained from the California poppy is a major advantage of this analgesic agent. A good night's sleep is critical for the body's healing.

You can learn more about the products Guy Chamberland develops for pain relief, and pain-associated insomnia, by visiting his website at www.guy-chamberland-herbalist.com. From this website you will find links to the different product brands that are based on his research.

Chapter 5
MANAGEMENT OF SPASMS-CRAMPS

This chapter introduces the reader to antispasmodic herbs and to those Guy Chamberland used and still uses to reduce the leg cramps and back muscle spasms from a chronic disc hernia.

Licorice (liquorice) (*Glycyrrhiza glabra*) is not as well-known in western herbology for its antispasmodic effects in pain management. It is better known for its anti-inflammatory effects on the gastrointestinal tract and as an expectorant. This plant is found in the *Eclectic Materia Medica*, but it had no recognized use in the treatment of pain conditions (Felter 1922). The active plant part is the dried rhizome. The rhizome has been used externally for its anti-inflammatory properties. An infusion made from 1 to 1.5 grams of the dried rhizome in 150 ml of boiling water is the common daily dose. According to WHO (1999), 5 to 15 grams of the dried plant material can be taken daily, and this corresponds to 200-800 mg of glycyrrhizin.

It has been used in Traditional Chinese medicine (TCM) for its antispasmodic activity. In fact it is commonly used in TCM in combination with White Peony for treating many types of muscle spasms, including those of the lower limbs. Its spasmolytic activity has been demonstrated in animals (WHO 1999).

Skullcap (*Scutellaria lateriflora*) (sometimes spelled Scullcap), also known as Virginia Skullcap and Helmet flower, is a well know anxiolytic and sedative herb. The active plant part is the dried aerial parts. It is known for its anticonvulsant, sedative, and antispasmodic properties. Guy Chamberland commonly uses this herb as an antispasmodic for muscle spasms and cramping and calmative in cases of anxiety. It is used in several products he developed for menstrual pain.

Typical doses range from infusion of 1 to 2 grams of the dried herb taken 3 times a day to equivalent amounts in the form of extracts or tinctures. You can take 0.25 to 12 grams of the dried herb top per day.

According to the *Eclectic Materia Medica* (Felter 1922), Skullcap is calmative to the nervous and muscular systems. Felter (1922) described it as able to control nervous irritability and muscular incoordination, thereby providing rest and allowing sleep, and it was described as a remedy for insomnia due to worry, nervous irritability or nervous excitability. It was used to control muscular twitching and tremors. Similar properties were described in the *American Materia Medica*, including the ability of the herb to induce a quiet and restful sleep via its action on the nervous system (Ellingwood & Lloyd 1919).

Skullcap was traditionally used as a nerve tonic and sedative including for its use in the treatment of epilepsy, grand mal, hysteria and nervous conditions (van Wyk & Wink 2010). According to Culbreth (1927), it was used as a nervine and antispasmodic medicine in the early 1900's and the *Manual of Materia Medica* lists the following pain associated conditions where it was used: spasms, muscular twitching, and neuralgia. Today it is widely used for treating tension, anxiety and insomnia as well as a visceral relaxant / antispasmodic for muscular cramps.

Valerian (*Valeriana officinalis*), also known as **Common Valerian**, is a popular sleep remedy. The active parts of the plant are the rhizomes and roots, and remedies made from these are considered sedatives (tranquilizers).

It is a mild sedative and sleep-promoting agent and has been used as an alternative to pharmaceutical sedatives, such as benzodiazepines in the treatment of nervous excitation and anxiety-induced sleep disturbances (WHO 1999). Its use as a sleep aid has been demonstrated in clinical trials. According to van Wyk & Wink (2010), it is recognized as a non-addictive tranquilizer for the treatment of restlessness, sleeplessness, minor nervous conditions, symptoms of menopause, and anxiety associated with premenstrual syndrome, and it has been traditionally used as supportive treatment for gastrointestinal pain and spastic colitis. Based on its antispasmodic properties, it has been used as an adjuvant in spasmolytic states of smooth muscle and gastrointestinal pains of nervous origin (WHO 1999).

In the early 1900's, it was listed as a medicine in the *American* and *Eclectic Materia Medica* and used for the following pain associated conditions: as an anodyne, nervine, antispasmodic (Culbreth 1927). Culbreth (1927) stated that when used continuously it could produce "melancholia". According to Marles et al (2000), this plant was used for multiple medical purposes by the Native Americans but none were for treating pain. The *Eclectic Materia Medica* described this plant as cerebral and spinal stimulant and a good calmative for nervousness (Felter 1922). The *American Materia Medica* (Ellingwood & Lloyd 1919) viewed the plant as a non-narcotic, recognized it as a nervine, and listed the following indications: hysterical conditions, nervous excitement, etc.

Doses range from 2 to 10 grams of the dried root daily taken in doses of 2 to 3 grams 1 to 5 times a day. Guy Chamberland used this herbal agent as a replacement for the prescribed muscle relaxant during the first two years but then switched to Scullcap. He found that Scullcap was a more powerful antispasmodic. Many people do not like using Valerian because of its odor so Scullcap is a great and superior alternative.

White Peony (*Paeonia lactiflora*) is an herb commonly used in India and Asia for its analgesic, anti-inflammatory and antispasmodic properties (van Wyk & Wink 2010; WHO 1999; Bone 1996). According to Bone 1996, it relieves spasms and is used in the treatment of muscle cramping and dysmenorrhoea. Experimental studies demonstrated these pharmacological properties.

It has been traditionally used in the treatment of headache, amenorrhea, dysmenorrhoea, and pain in the chest and abdomen, as well as lower limbs (e.g. spasms of the calf muscles) (WHO 1999). The active part of the plant that is traditionally used is the dried root. The doses range from 6 to 15 grams of the dried root per day.

Guy Chamberland uses both enteric coated tablets and capsules of extracts of Scullcap as an antispasmodic agent. Two tablets or capsules of Scullcap are effectively used for treating muscle spasms or cramps. People have different sensitivities to the effects of this herb so be careful when using it for the first time. It was demonstrated in a clinical trial (Wolfson & Hoffmann 2003) that its sedative activity increases with increasing dosage. In some people, the drowsiness can be important so proceed carefully when using this herb during the day.

He found that the combined use of Devil's claw, California poppy plus Scullcap was very effective during periods of moderate or severe low back pain, with lower leg cramps, and back muscle spasms. Scullcap is taken three times a day because of its short duration of action. The short duration is not an issue because relief is usually obtained relatively fast. Some people consider short duration to be a problem because you need to take the product three times a day or more. He does not share this view because safety and efficacy is very important and Scullcap has a very good track record.

The combination of Licorice with White Peony could be an option for people that do not obtain adequate relief from Scullcap or Valerian.

You can learn more about the products Guy Chamberland develops for pain relief, and pain-associated insomnia, by visiting his website at www.guy-chamberland-herbalist.com. From this website you will find links to the different product brands that are based on his research.

Chapter 6
MANAGEMENT OF INSOMNIA

This chapter introduces the reader to herbs used for the treatment of insomnia. There are many causes of insomnia and choices for treating each condition. This book is dedicated to pain and living with pain therefore this chapter will only discuss the treatment of pain-associated insomnia. In 2007, Guy Chamberland would have liked to know what he does today. The many sleepless nights due to pain would not have occurred.

California poppy (*Eschscholzia californica*) is an herb traditionally used in North America for its analgesic, hypnotic and sedative properties. The active part of the plant is the dried aerial parts. It has been traditionally used to treat sleeplessness (e.g. insomnia) in adults and children, anxiety, minor nervous disturbances, neuralgic pains, toothaches, and liver and gallbladder complaints (van Wyk & Wink 2010). You can read about its pain relief properties in the chapter on analgesic herbs.

You may experience drowsiness when taking this herb. You may also develop tolerance to the sensation of drowsiness after taking several doses of of this herb; however, in general you should continue to benefit from the hypnotic (e.g. sleep aid) effects of the herb. In general, people do not have a next-morning residual drowsiness when using this herb as a sleep aid. Also, there are no reports of reduced concentration or reduced motor coordination.

Experimental studies confirmed the sedative/hypnotic pharmacological properties of California poppy (Gafner et al 2006; Rolland et al 2001). According to other studies, the time it takes to fall asleep is reduced and the sleep quality is improved.

There is no known dependence or addiction to California poppy. This is why it is not classified as a narcotic or controlled drug.

Doses range from 0.5 to 3 grams per day of the dried herb.

Corydalis (*Corydalis yanhusuo*) is an herb used in traditional Chinese medicine for its analgesic activity and sedative activities (Bone 1996). These activities have been demonstrated experimentally and it used in the treatment of insomnia. The active part of the plant is the rhizome. Doses range from 5 to 10 grams of the dried rhizome per day.

Hops (*Humulus lupulus*) have been shown to possess sedative and hypnotic effects. Traditionally, this herb has been used for relaxation, anxiety, and sedation, and to treat insomnia. The Cherokee Natives used hops as a sedative and analgesic. In traditional Chinese medicine, hops are used to treat insomnia and restlessness. Several clinical studies have examined the use of Hops in combination with Valerian (*Valeriana officinalis*) for the treatment of sleep disturbances. The active part of the plant is the strobili. Doses range from 0.5 to 6 grams per day, taken before bedtime.

Guy Chamberland has developed sleep aid products containing the combination of Hops with California poppy. These combinations were found to be very good for treating insomnia. Based on the analgesic properties of both herbs, this combination is useful as a sleep aid for cases of mild-to-moderate night pain. This combination has not been found to affect alertness and its sedative effects occur within 15 to 30 minutes after intake.

Skullcap (*Scutellaria lateriflora*) (sometimes spelled Scullcap), also known as Virginia Skullcap and Helmet flower, is a well know anxiolytic and sedative herb. The active plant part is the dried aerial parts. It is known for its anticonvulsant, sedative, and antispasmodic properties. It should not be mistaken for its Asian sister (a well known Chinese herb) (Baical Skullcap / *Scutellaria baicalensis*) which are known for their anti-inflammatory, anti-allergic and circulatory properties.

Native Americans used Marsh Skullcap (*Scutellaria galericulata*) as a remedy for ulcers and fever (Marles et al 2000). According to these authors, an extract of Marsh Skullcap showed no sedative or antispasmodic effects. According to the *Eclectic Materia Medica* (Felter 1922), Skullcap is calmative to the nervous and muscular systems. Felter (1922) described it as able to control nervous irritability and muscular incoordination, thereby providing rest and allowing sleep, and it was described as a remedy for insomnia due to worry, nervous irritability or nervous excitability. It was used to control muscular twitching and tremors. Similar properties were described in the *American Materia Medica*, including the ability of the herb to induce a quiet and restful sleep via its action on the nervous system (Ellingwood & Lloyd 1919).

Virginia Skullcap was traditionally used as a nerve tonic and sedative including for its use in the treatment of epilepsy, grand mal, hysteria and nervous conditions (van Wyk & Wink 2010). According to Culbreth (1927), it was used as a nervine and antispasmodic medicine in the early 1900's and the *Manual of Materia Medica* lists the following pain associated conditions where it was used: spasms, muscular twitching, and neuralgia. Today it is widely used for treating tension, anxiety and insomnia as well as a visceral relaxant / antispasmodic for muscular cramps.

Typical doses range from infusion of 1 to 2 grams of the dried herb taken 3 times a day to equivalent amounts in the form of extracts or tinctures. You can take 0.25 to 12 grams of the dried herb top per day.

Valerian (*Valeriana officinalis*), also known as **Common Valerian**, is a popular sleep remedy. It has been used as a sedative and anxiolytic for more than 2,000 years (Natural Standard database). The active parts of the plant are the rhizomes and roots, and remedies made from these are considered sedatives (tranquilizers). It is a mild sedative and sleep-promoting agent and has been used as an alternative to pharmaceutical sedatives, such as benzodiazepines in the treatment of nervous excitation and anxiety-induced sleep disturbances (WHO 1999). Its use as a sleep aid has been demonstrated in clinical trials. The results of these studies suggest that its benefits are observed after several days of repeated use and not after a single dose. Progressive effects are observed over several weeks. Studies have also shown that it is more effective in combination with herbs like Hops.

According to van Wyk & Wink (2010), it is recognized as a non-addictive tranquilizer for the treatment of restlessness, sleeplessness, minor nervous conditions, symptoms of menopause, and anxiety associated with premenstrual syndrome, and it has been traditionally used as supportive treatment for gastrointestinal pain and spastic colitis. Based on its antispasmodic properties, it has been used as an adjuvant in spasmolytic states of smooth muscle and gastrointestinal pains of nervous origin (WHO 1999).

Other herbs, such as **Lemon balm** (*Melissa officinalis*) and **Passion flower** (*Passiflora incarnata*) also have a long history of use in the treatment of insomnia. Some of these herbs, used alone or in combination, are very good choices for restlessness or insomnia due to mental stress. Guy Chamberland has not used these other herbs for treating pain-associated insomnia. His preferred herbs for insomnia have been California poppy, Hops and Scullcap. His studies have found that the combination of California poppy with Scullcap is very good for the treatment of anxiety-related insomnia but this topic will be addressed in his next book.

For pain-associated insomnia, he uses California poppy as the key therapeutic ingredient. This herb is both analgesic and sedative-hypnotic so it is ideal for this type of condition. The dose level of each herbal agent is critical when creating a strong formulation. For mild-to-moderate pain, the combination of California poppy with Hops usually provides sufficient analgesia and sedation to help the patient fall asleep. In the case of California poppy, his studies demonstrated that the sedative-hypnotic effect is dose-dependent. When combined with dried strobile of Hops, the sedative-hypnotic effect is even stronger. However, his studies demonstrated that there was a lower limit where the herbs no longer provide sedative-hypnotic benefits to the patient. When the dosages are well balanced, the sedative activity is usually felt 15 to 30 minutes after intake. Therefore, it is important to take the product 15 to 30 minutes before bedtime.

For moderate-to-severe pain, the combination of California poppy with Devil's claw is a better alternative. An effective product must still provide an adequate level of sedative activity. However, the patient usually requires more pain relief therefore it is important to add anti-inflammatory agents to the formulation. Clinical research performed by multiple teams has established the critical role of COX (cyclooxygenase) inhibitors in achieving acute pain relief. A natural herbal agent with COX-2 inhibition is Devil's claw. When used alone and at the correct dosage, it has been shown to provide adequate pain relief. It provides even better pain relief when used in combination with California poppy. Guy Chamberland developed products using these two herbal ingredients as a remedy for night pain.

From 2007 to 2008, he had many sleepless nights due to night pain. Since 2009, he deals with night pain by using either California poppy combined with Hops or California poppy combined with Devil's claw. The deciding factor is the level of pain and the use is according to what is described in the above paragraphs.

You can learn more about the products Guy Chamberland develops for pain relief, and pain-associated insomnia, by visiting his website at www.guy-chamberland-herbalist.com. From this website you will find links to the different product brands that are based on his research.

WORKS CITED

Allaert et al 1992. Allaert, F. A., Vin, F., and Levardon, M. *Comparative study of the effectiveness of continuous or intermittent courses of a phlebotonic drug on venous disorders disclosed or aggravated by oral, estrogen-progesterone contraceptives.* Phlebologie. 1992; 45(2):167-173.

Bone 1996. K Bone, *Clinical applications of Ayurvedic and Chinese herbs.* Phytotherapy Press, Australia, 1996.

Borrelli, F., Izzo, A. A., and Ernst, E. *Pharmacological effects of Cimicifuga racemosa.* Life Sci. 7-25-2003;73(10):1215-1229.

Briese et al 2007. Briese, V., Stammwitz, U., Friede, M., and Henneicke-von Zepelin, H. H. *Black cohosh with or without St. John's wort for symptom-specific climacteric treatment-results of a large-scale, controlled, observational study.* Maturitas 8-20-2007;57(4):405-414.

Culbreth 1927. D M R Culbreth, *A Manual of Materia Medica and Pharmacology.* Lea & Febiger, Philadelphia, 1927.

Dugoua et al 2006. Dugoua, J. J., Seely, D., Perri, D., Koren, G., and Mills, E. *Safety and efficacy of black cohosh (Cimicifuga racemosa) during pregnancy and lactation.* Can J Clin Pharmacol 2006;13(3):e257-e261.

Ellingwood & Lloyd 1919. Ellingwood F and Lloyd J U, *American Materia Medica, Therapeutics and Pharmacognosy.* Eclectic Medical Publications, Cincinnati, Ohio 1919.

Felter 1922. *The Eclectic Materia Medica, Pharmacology and Therapeutics.* Eclectic Medical Publications, Cincinnati, Ohio 1922.

Frank and Unger 2006. Frank, A. and Unger, M. *Analysis of frankincense from various Boswellia species with inhibitory activity on human drug metabolising cytochrome P450 enzymes using liquid chromatography mass spectrometry after automated on-line extraction.* J Chromatogr A 4-21-2006; 1112(1-2):255-262.

Gafner S et al 2006. Gafner S, Dietz BM, McPhail KL, Scott IM et al. *Alkaloids from Eschscholzia californica and their capacity to inhibit binding of [³H]8-hydroxy-2-(di-N-propylamino)tetralin to 5-HT$_{1A}$ receptors in vitro.* J Nat Prod 2006, 69, 432-435.

Grieve M 1971. Mrs. M Grieve. *A modern herbal: The medicinal, culinary, cosmetic and economic properties, cultivation and folk-lore of herbs, grasses, fungi, shrubs and trees with all their modern scientific uses.* Volumes I and II. Dover Publication, Inc, New York. 1971.

Health Canada. Monographs prepared by the Natural Health Products Directorate, Health Canada. http://webprod.hc-sc.gc.ca/nhpid-bdipsn/monosReq.do?lang=eng ; Accessed 2011.

Kiela et al 2005. Kiela, P. R., Midura, A. J., Kuscuoglu, N., Jolad, S. D., Solyom, A. M., Besselsen, D. G., Timmermann, B. N., and Ghishan, F. K. *Effects of Boswellia serrata in mouse models of chemically induced colitis.* Am J Physiol Gastrointest.Liver Physiol 2005;288(4):G798-G808.

Lupu et al 2003. Lupu, R., Mehmi, I., Atlas, E., Tsai, M. S., Pisha, E., Oketch-Rabah, H. A., Nuntanakorn, P., Kennelly, E. J., and Kronenberg, F. *Black cohosh, a menopausal remedy, does not have estrogenic activity and does not promote breast cancer cell growth.* Int J Oncol. 2003;23(5):1407-1412.

Mahady et al 2008. Mahady, G. B., Low, Dog T., Barrett, M. L., Chavez, M. L., Gardiner, P., Ko, R., Marles, R. J., Pellicore, L. S., Giancaspro, G. I., and Sarma, D. N. *United States Pharmacopeia review of the black cohosh case reports of hepatotoxicity.* Menopause. 2008;15(4 Pt 1):628-638.

Marles et al 2000. Marles RJ, Clavelle C, Monteleone L, Tays N and Burns D, *Aboriginal plant use in Canada's Northwest Boreal Forest*, Natural Resources Canada, UBC Press, Vancouver 2000.

Moore et al 2003. Moore A, Edwards J, Barden J et McQuay H. *Bandolier's Little Book of Pain.* Oxford University Press, 2003.

Natural Standard database. *Evidence-based Systematic Reviews of herbs* by the Natural Standard Research Collaboration. Copyright ® 2011. www.natural standard.com. Accessed 2011.

Reame et al 2008. Reame, N. E., Lukacs, J. L., Padmanabhan, V., Eyvazzadeh, A. D., Smith, Y. R., and Zubieta, J. K. *Black cohosh has central opioid activity in postmenopausal women: evidence from naloxone blockade and positron emission tomography neuroimaging.* Menopause. 2008; 15(5):832-840.

Rolland A et al 2001. Rolland A, Fleurentin J, Lanhers MC et al. *Neurophysiological effects of an extract of Escholzia californica Cham (Papaveraceae).* Phytother. Res. 2001; 15:377-381.

Sarris J et Wardle J 2010. Sarris J et Wardle J. *Clinical naturopathy: an evidence-based guide to practice.* Churchill Livingstone, Elsevier. 2010.

Seidlova-Wuttke et al 2003. Seidlova-Wuttke, D., Hesse, O., Jarry, H., Christoffel, V., Spengler, B., Becker, T., and Wuttke, W. *Evidence for selective estrogen receptor modulator activity in a black cohosh (Cimicifuga racemosa) extract: comparison with estradiol-17beta.* Eur.J Endocrinol. 2003;149(4): 351-362.

van Wyk & Wink 2010. BE van Wyk and M Wink, *Medicinal Plants of the World*, Timber Press, 2010.

Viereck et al 2005. Viereck, V., Grundker, C., Friess, S. C., Frosch, K. H., Raddatz, D., Schoppet, M., Nisslein, T., Emons, G., and Hofbauer, L. C. *Isopropanolic extract of black cohosh stimulates osteoprotegerin production by human osteoblasts.* J Bone Miner. Res 2005;20(11):2036-2043.

WHO (1999). World Health Organization, Geneva. *WHO monographs on selected medicinal plants.* Volume 1, 1999.

Wolfson & Hoffmann 2003. P. Wolfson and DL Hoffmann. *An investigation into the efficacy of Scutellaria lateriflora in healthy volunteers.* Altern Ther Health Med 2003;9(2):74-78.

ABOUT THE AUTHOR

GUY CHAMBERLAND, *M.Sc., Ph.D., Master Herbalist*, is a retired drug development specialist that spent over 15 years in the pharmaceutical industry bringing new products from discovery to *first in human* clinical trials and then to the market. He obtained a Master's of Science and Doctorate (PhD) degree in the biomedical sciences (field of toxicology). Chamberland developed an expertise in drug safety and regulatory affairs while working in the pharmaceutical and biotechnology industries.

Chamberland has completed training as a natural health practitioner, bioenergetics practitioner, chartered herbalist, in herbal prescriptions, and performed clinical research to obtain the degree of Master Herbalist. Through his continued research in herbal science, he has become an expert in herbal pain management.

He founded the company called CuraPhyte Technologies. You can visit the websites at www.curaphyte.com and www.enteriphyte.com. You can reach Chamberland at gchamberland@ curaphyte.ca.

Chamberland is currently working on his next book entitled *Scientific Look at Herbal Remedies: Is there more than Traditional Evidence*?